Dedicated to
Teachers
and
the Art
of Teaching.

**Paperback ISBN:** 979-8-9861693-0-9
**E-book ISBN:** 979-8-9861693-2-3

# Exercise.

# Why?

**(Mindful thoughts of a Personal Trainer)**

**Jeff Shammah**

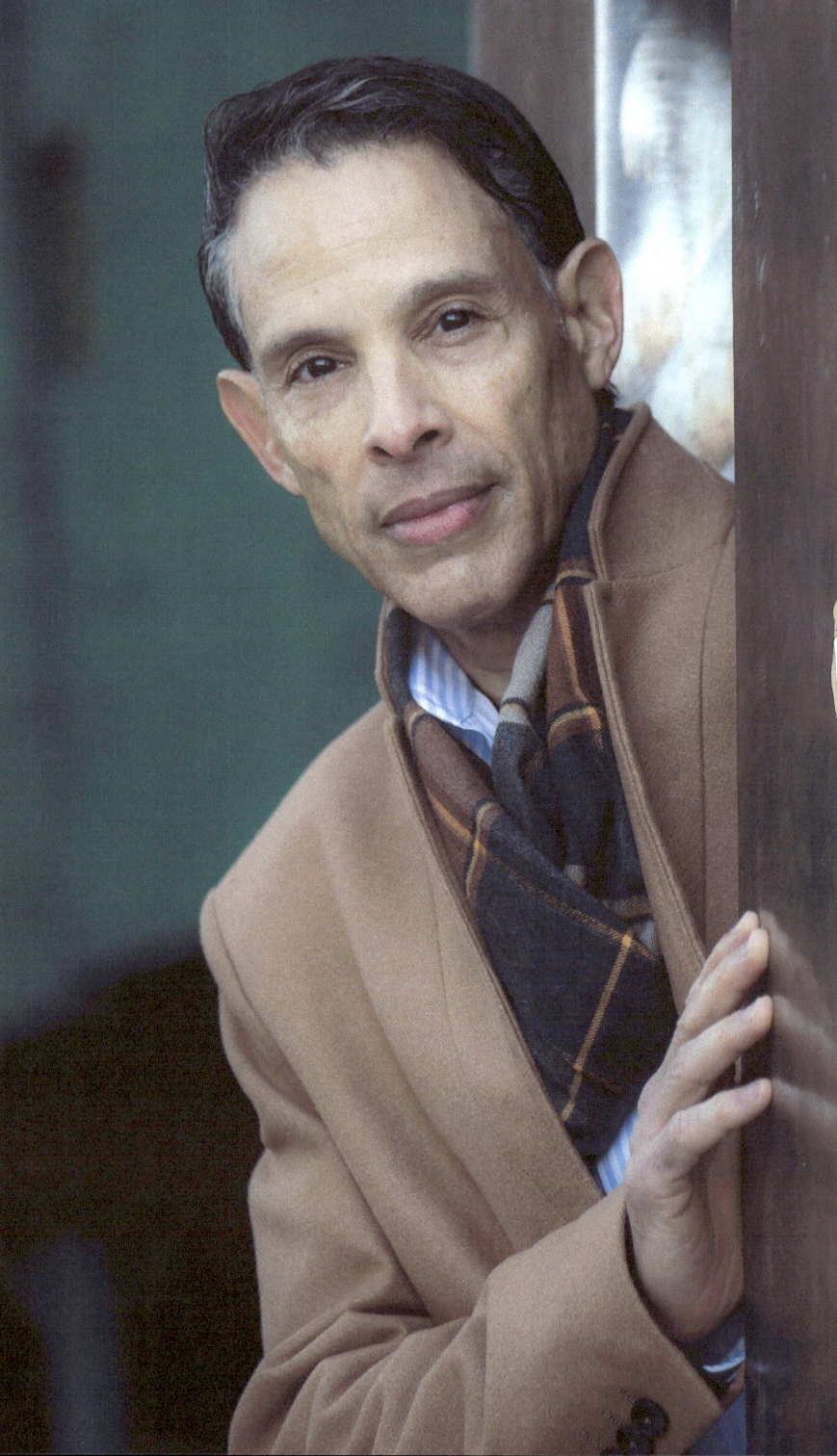

# This book is meant to be:

Short, Simple and Universal.

# Think for oneself...

It will not give out answers!
It is an outline only.

# It will...

'romote and provoke individuals to **think** for themselves and seek out answers by asking questions.

# It is:

- A general guide book
- A reference tool
- Philosophical
- Non-specific
- **Timeless**

# Universal Principles

Guiding principles that we can use towards exercise throughout our lives. Ideas and thoughts that are flexible and maleable to change as we change.

**Discipline** is the primary thing we all need to apply in order to grow as human beings and to manage difficult times.

**Exercise** is one of the most basic ways of achieving and re-enforcing Discipline.

# Exercise.
## Why?

Exercise is one of
the most important and basic forms
of **"Self Discovery."**
A process of **Experiencing** ourselves.

# 1. The Mind

A child's early mental development is through physical movement: **Motor skills** (brain development.)

Exercises that involve both mind and body working in unison, have longer lasting and farther reaching benefits, than just mental exercises alone.

As a child learns to sit, crawl and walk, its brain develops through physical activity and experience, long before it can either read or write.

Illnesses such as Dementia-Alzheimer's may be slowed or its progression stopped through continued preventative exercises involving the mind and body in new and challenging ways.

# 2. The Body

Physical fitness is necessary so that the body (the soldier) is able to carry out the orders of the mind (the General). In all the forms that life demands of us.

Longevity requires physical capability in order to maintain **Independence** as we age.

# 3. The Spirit/Emotional Self

Feelings of self worth, self confidence are strengthened and reinforced through exercise. Combating depression and the release of anger (venting system) through sweat are all **natural side effects of exercising.**

Do we really make our best contributions to society while we are young? Or is the **"unnecessarily fast"** deterioration of our minds, body and spirit to blame?

A lack of consistent exercise:
*"If you don't use it, you lose it."* may be the true deterrent that keeps us from being consistent contributers to Life!

# One Body:

The same body studied by all health professionals but with different focuses.

We need to give it the **same respect and reverence through exercise** that we do when we see our doctors.

This wonderous machine requires the same **detail, choice and order** of treatment (exercise) that we give it when we choose our health professionals to combat and prevent illness.

**An exercise prescription** that evolves and changes with us as we age.

# Read and Ponder or Meditate on Each

The following are ideas, phrases and subjects that will help in personalizing your exercise prescription.

1. One size does **not** fit all

2. Balanced approach

3. Practice does **not** make perfect

4. Bring the right problem to the right person

5. Recuperation

6. Athletes

7. As we age it is important that we learn to train **smarter not** necessarily **harder.**

8. Meditation

9. Wisdom is the proper use of experience

10. Personal Training

# 1. One size does not fit all

As convenient as it may be or sound, there will never be one form or way to exercise, that is correct for everyone.

We all need to maintain our bodies but the **type, intensity, duration** and **frequency** will vary from person to person.

These variables will not only need **adjusting daily, weekly, and yearly,** but so will our needs as we age.

Instead of forcing ourselves to fit, we should look forward to and welcome change and diversity, and the opportunity it will give us to get to know our **new** selves as we evolve through life.

Exercise will always be subject to fads or trends but in the end it is still exercise with a "shiny new suit."

Take the time to find out what works for you and be open to change when necessary.

This idea is not just applicable to exercise but to **nutrition** and **sleep** as well.

# 2. Balanced approach

When we exercise, it is important to maintain a balanced approach when addressing the bodies various physical needs, in order to be "physically fit."

**Muscular strength, muscular endurance, flexibility, balance, coordination, agility** and **speed** are areas that we will need to become proficient at, in order to properly function physically in life.

These basic building blocks will also contribute to the foundation towards spiritual health.

**A sound mind + sound body = spirit** are the prerequisites that give birth to a sound spirit. Always use a **holistic approach** when it comes to good health. **Integration** and a **complimentative** approach to **nutrition, exercise** and **sleep,** will help us achieve **balance.**

*An exercise program should be composed of equal parts **free compound movement** and **isolated movements.** They compliment one another **(Yin/Yang).** And when necessary an emphasis on an area **(therapy)** until imbalance is corrected.

Then a gradual return to a more well rounded routine to help prevent future health problems.

# 3. Practice...
## does not make Perfect

Only correct practice leads towards improvement. If we repeat something over and over incorrectly, it will only reinforce imperfection.

The same way that we choose our health professionals according to the alignment of our illness and their area of specialization, we need to apply the same logic towards exercise.

What do we need or want to accomplish or achieve through exercise?

Which health professional is specifically schooled in and best qualified to teach us and answer our questions?

We need to be patient and progressive in our learning. **More** of anything **does not necessarily** translate into **better. It is the willingness to practice through Trial and Error and make continuous adjustments as we learn, that leads towards Self Knowledge.**

When beginning and throughout our exercise journey, it is important that we **think** about and apply a progressive approach to exercising.

**What, How, When, How Intense, How Long** and **How Frequent.**

We will not improve or achieve our goals, if our approach to exercise is **mindless.**

# It does matter!

# 4. Bring the right problem to the right person

The **root** or cause of a physical imbalance must first be identified in order to eliminate **chronic pain.**

This requires an initial search and some trial and error **as opposed to a quick fix solution.**

In doing so we need to maintain an open mind in choosing our health professionals.

As well trained and qualified they may be in their field of expertise, if it does not align with the root of the problem, the answer will not be found.

Work with health professionals who are specifically qualified and schooled in your area of need.

# 5. Recuperation

Whether mental, physical or emotional, recuperation is the key to results. Exercise is an intentional stress placed on the mind, body and spirit.

This stress causes a reaction by the body that leads to an adaptation over time, and change of some kind.

In order for this stress, adaptation and change to lead towards positive results, we must leave adequate time for recuperation between exercise sessions.

**Exercise + Nutrition + Sleep = Results**

* The continued effort to properly balance out these three areas will lead to **positive results.**

* An emphasis on one over the other "unless when needed" will lead to imbalance and **negative results.**

# 6. Athletes

## There is a difference between exercising and **understanding** exercise.

Often as athletes we are given exercises to do, and we perform them in an obedient disciplined fashion without question. These exercises are properly aligned with the needs of the given sport in order to compete successfully.

**But,** understanding the physiological processes that are going on in the body, and the future negative ramifications of these exercises through repetitive movement over long periods of time, are rarely discussed. This often leads to many future health problems in the aging and retired athlete.

The athlete is often left in the dark as how to properly exercise for **well rounded general fitness,** as opposed to a sport.

When we do not have a basic fundamental understanding of how the body works it can have a profound effect on an athlete's mental, physical and emotional well being.

## Sample questions to ask oneself:

- Exercise after retirement?
- How do I fix repetitive movement or overuse injuries?
- Teaching: how to teach less physically gifted individuals?
- Exercising for mental and emotional health after retirement?

# 7. As we age it is important that we learn to train <u>smarter</u> not necessarily <u>harder</u>.

Youth is a time for experimentation in all areas of our lives. These lessons learned are there to serve us as we age.

Exercise is no different. The cool, fun, trendy exercises and one size fits all programs served a purpose in our initial experience with exercise. But, as we age our genetic differences, injuries, health issues and needs, change from one person to another.

It therefore becomes very important to evolve into an **Individual Health Prescription.**

Exercise just for the sake of exercise, is no longer adequate and is potentially dangerous.

Your exercise routine should address **your personal individual needs.**

There should be a plan based on mindful thought, that is adjustable and flexible to your individual needs, on any given day and moment, that continues to evolve over time.

**We need to connect the dots as we age, of our life's Experiences and Lessons, in order to see our:**

## Individual Picture!

# 8. Meditation

Meditative practice on our individual self and body helps us to understand our relationship to each other and our place in the universe.

The human body is a wonderous and complex miniature product (micro-cosm) of the much larger and awe inspiring universe (macro-cosm).

Through exercise, for which:

## "Its Simplicity is its Genius"

Anyone can begin this conversation with, and continued dialogue, using ones own body, through the most basic formative way of learning: **Motor Skills.** Once this foundation has been laid, it is then possible to reach ones individual potential.

The greater the understanding of oneself, the more secure our relationship will be to others. Recognizing how much we all have in common: **the basis for security,** as opposed to not: **the basis for insecurity.**

This commonality allows us to see all forms of exercise as more the same rather than different.

**Therefore providing an open mind to learning new things, change, and allowing a flexible approach to exercise that evolves with us as we age.**

# 9. Wisdom is the proper use of experience.

If we approach our exercise routine using our past experiences, and overall knowledge of ourselves, it will serve to help us make wiser choices.

If we dogmatically repeat and refuse to listen to our bodies, then:

**some form of illness or injury will occur and re-occur until we stop and change.**

# 10. Personal Training

Personal training is one of the best opportunities to effect change, quite simply, because of its frequency. A personal trainer will normally see an individual or individuals 1 to 3x per week (excluding holidays and vacations), all year long.

Versus, a once a year visit to the doctor, for a general checkup or 6 to 8 weeks of physical therapy to recuperate from an injury.

Regardless of how extraordinary these health professionals are, they just don't have or spend, the amount of time with an individual necessary, to effect **preventative** or **life changing habits.**

The attention and frequency given to an individual during a one-to-one exercise session, affords the time to explore that persons physical, mental and spiritual needs.

This allows overtime for the development of a **personal exercise prescription,** as opposed to a one size fits all approach.

Adjusting an individuals exercise: **intensity, duration** and **frequency** can be monitored in a progressive manner, and adapted at any given session for **that day's needs, not** a chart with pre-planned exercises.

There are many ways to effectively use a personal trainer, that can offset cost and available time.

**Examples:**

- 1-3x per week
- 1x per month check up
- 1x every three months, session, to discuss changes and upgrades to an existing routine.
- Sharing the hour with 1 or 2 other individuals, to lower your individual cost.

**The most important factor is to take the time, to find a well schooled or accredited teacher, with the experience and patience, to guide you on this individual journey.**

There are many great teachers with a wide variety of skills, so this may include a bit of trial and error, in order to arrive at a clearer idea of what you may **need not necessarily want.**

# Hopefully, Helpful Thoughts and Suggestions

# Human Body
## "machine of forgiveness"

Except for those individuals who unfortunately and through no fault of their own, have been born with severe genetic defects, the human bodys capacity to regenerate, heal and forgive is truly amazing.

What I mean by forgive is its ability to function **despite** our continued **misuse, neglect,** and **overuse** of the **"best friend"** we take for granted, until we push it one time too many.

Because of its resilience and remarkable design, and an immune system with an enormous capacity to adapt, we too often ignore its **early cries for help and signals that how we are living our lives and treating our bodies is incorrect.**

We blame **age, momentary circumstances or ignorance,** rather than take responsibility for ignoring its needs.

In most cases when we finally breakdown mentally, emotionally or physically it rarely is due to any recent changes, but more often due to the body and its immune system, finally losing the battle it has been waging overtime on our behalf, and our refusal to acknowledge it and **change.**

## But there is hope!

In a relatively short amount of time the body can slowdown, stop and in cases reverse most of the damage done to it.

**If we are willing to change.**

Ultimately for:

**Youth:** develop good habits early on that will serve us later in life.

**Middle Age:** acknowledge the need for change, adaptation and flexibility.

**Older Age:** it truly is **"never too late"**

The body can and will improve at any age. Use wisdom and experience, to create an exercise prescription specific to your needs.

**The brain and body will respond to correct technique applied: Progressively, Consistently and Patiently.**

Results will follow.

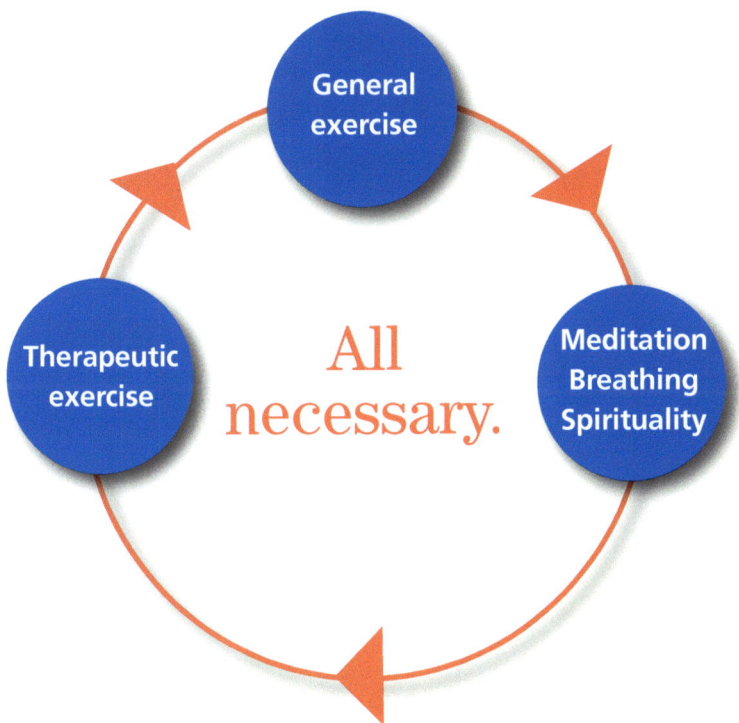

General
exercise

Meditation
Breathing
Spirituality

Therapeutic
exercise

All
necessary.

# All equally important.

**Placing the emphasis, at any given time,**

**on the area with the greatest deficiency.**

# Insurance
# and Supplements

**1.** We often purchase insurance first (encouraged to buy the most expensive) when we would be better off investing in:

**Nutrition, Exercise and Sleep.**

Then insurance **(just in case).**

**2.** We often purchase supplements first

**(rather than change or improve our eating habits)**

Then supplements **(if needed).**

**We need to restore the proper order and priority of these two in our lives.**

**Rather than take short cuts towards better health.**

# Process of
# Subtraction not Addition

All of these ideas may seem overwhelming at first. But, as we age we gain the experience and knowledge, to begin the process of eliminating that which has outlived its usefulness, and emphasize the few things that really matter to us.

**Thereby leaving more time for that which we need to do, and love to do.**

# Blessed with the Gift of Time...

In my **38 years** as a personal trainer, I have had the good fortune of maintaining relationships with clientele, for an average of **5 to 20 years** each.

I can only hope that I have been as good a teacher for them, as they have been for me.

Here are a few of my longest and continuing to date.

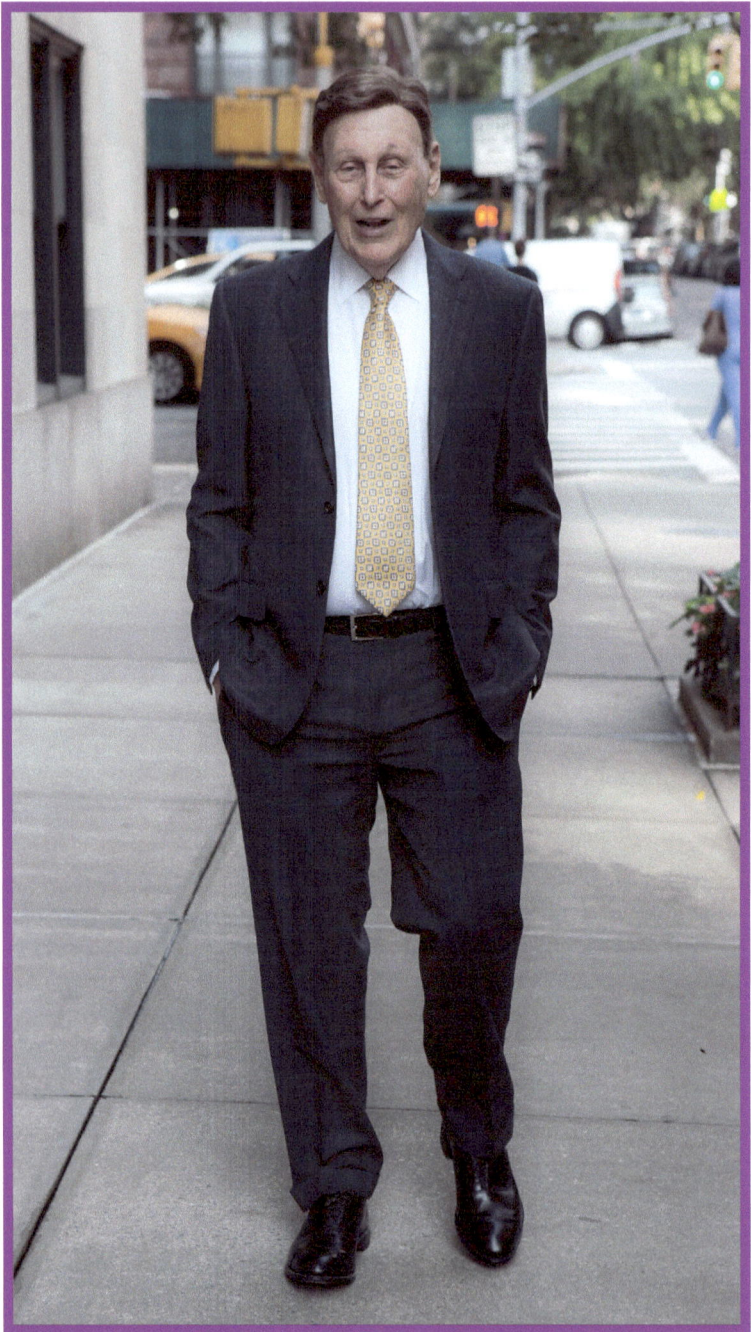

# Name: Gerald Modell
# Age: 87

Started his personal training with me at the age of 56.
We have been together for a total of **30 years
and counting...**

Businessman and owner of Modell Inc., he is still working
by choice, because as he puts it:

> *"I wish to remain productive and*
> *continue to contribute...*
> *because there is still much left to achieve!"*

**\*Special note and Memoriam to:**
**Paula Modell,** who I also had the honor of personally
training for **25 years.**

*I miss you.*

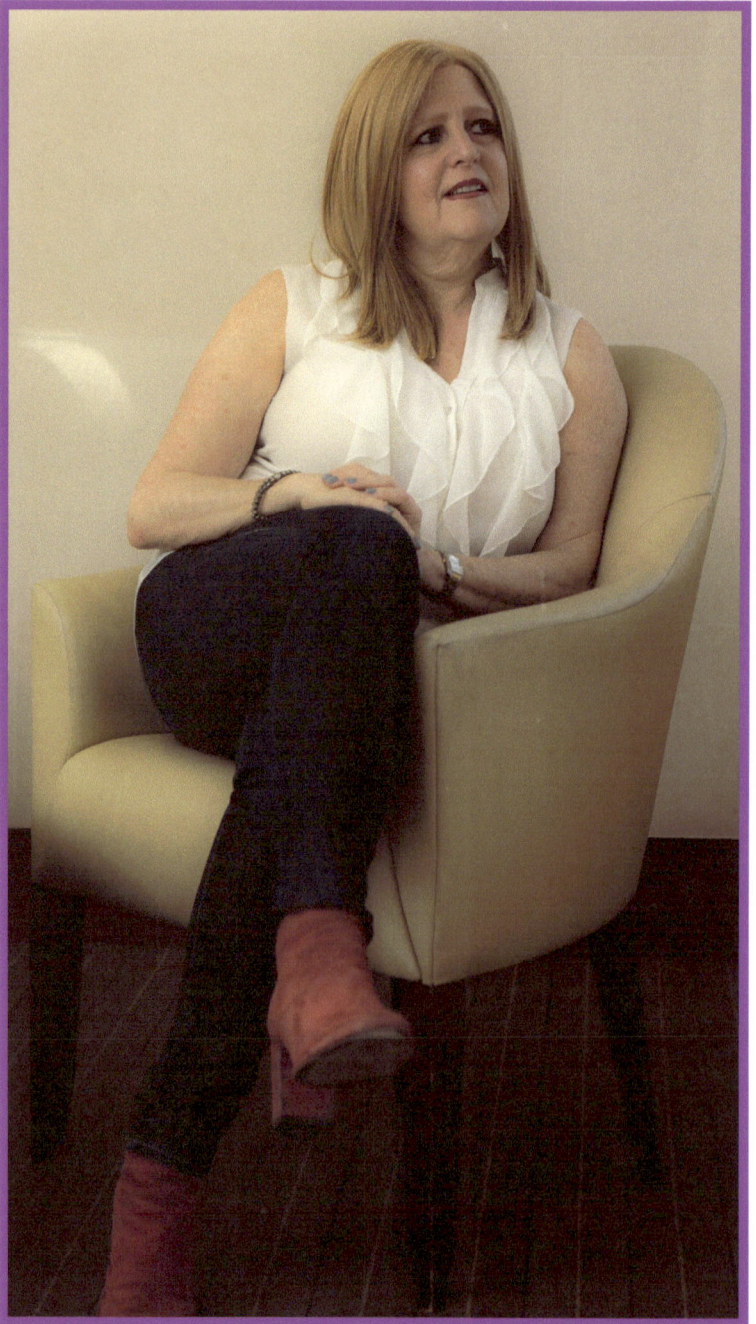

# Name: Elizabeth Beck
# Age: 59

Started her personal training with me at the age of 30. We have been together for a total of **29 years and counting...**

Liz Beck is an integrated marketing and communications specialist for a global public relations agency. She specializes in campaigns that engage consumers, reinforce differentiation and deliver business results.

Liz has made working out and movement a priority for nearly three decades. She's an avid scuba diver with more than 400 dives logged. She is also a runner and completed two New York City marathons. Pilates and strength training round out her fitness routine.

*"Exercise started as a way to stay in shape, and now it is crucial to my ability to stay active, healthy and strong."*

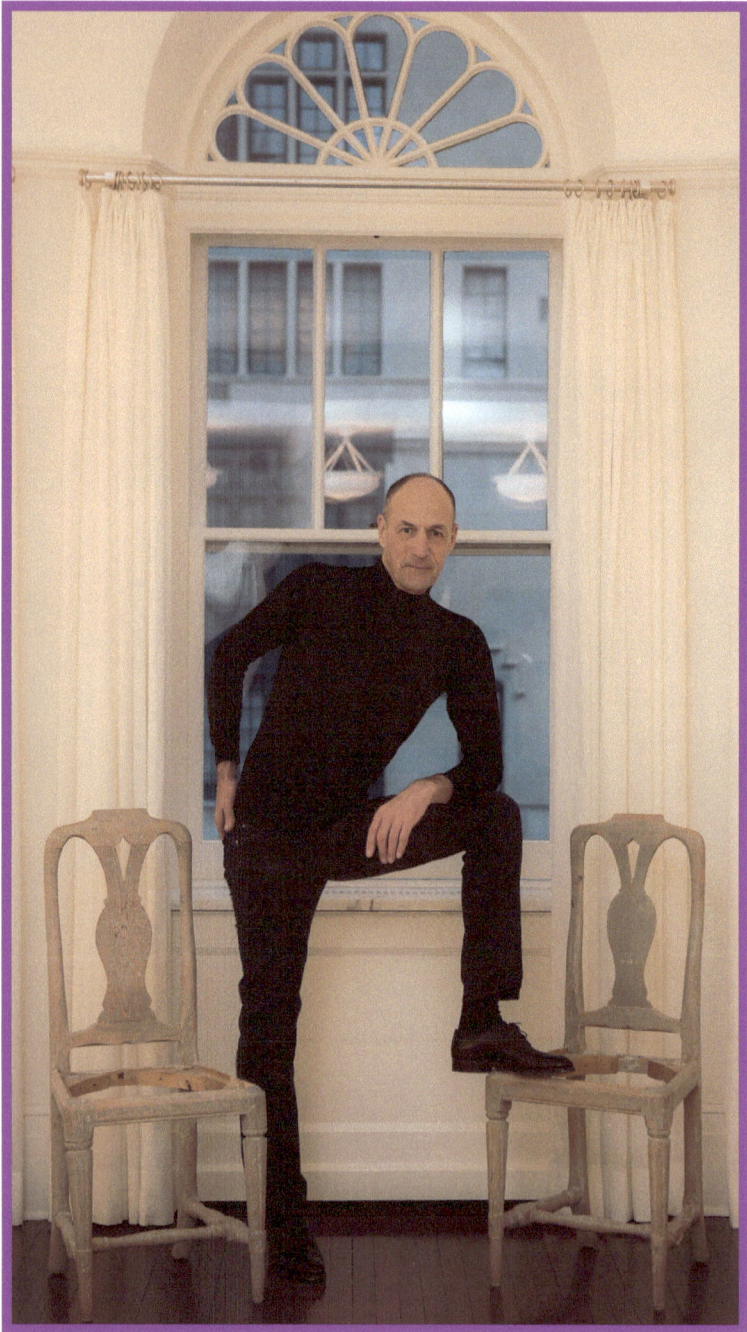

# Name: Anthony Dub
# Age: 70

Started his personal training with me at the age of 42. We have been together for a total of **28 years and counting...**

Tony is Chairman of Indigo Capital, LLC, a financial advisory firm based in New York City. Before forming Indigo Capital in 1997, he worked at Credit Suisse First Boston for 26 years, leading a number of departments including Investment Banking, Capital Markets, Mortgage Finance and Asset Finance.

Tony is an avid skier, having participated in expeditions to Alaska, Greenland and Iceland, which he still visits frequently, as he loves to "skin" up some far off mountain with an experienced guide and friends.

None of this would be possible without an active training program.

*"Life is short, and we should enjoy every day and try to make whatever contribution we can to make the world a better place."*

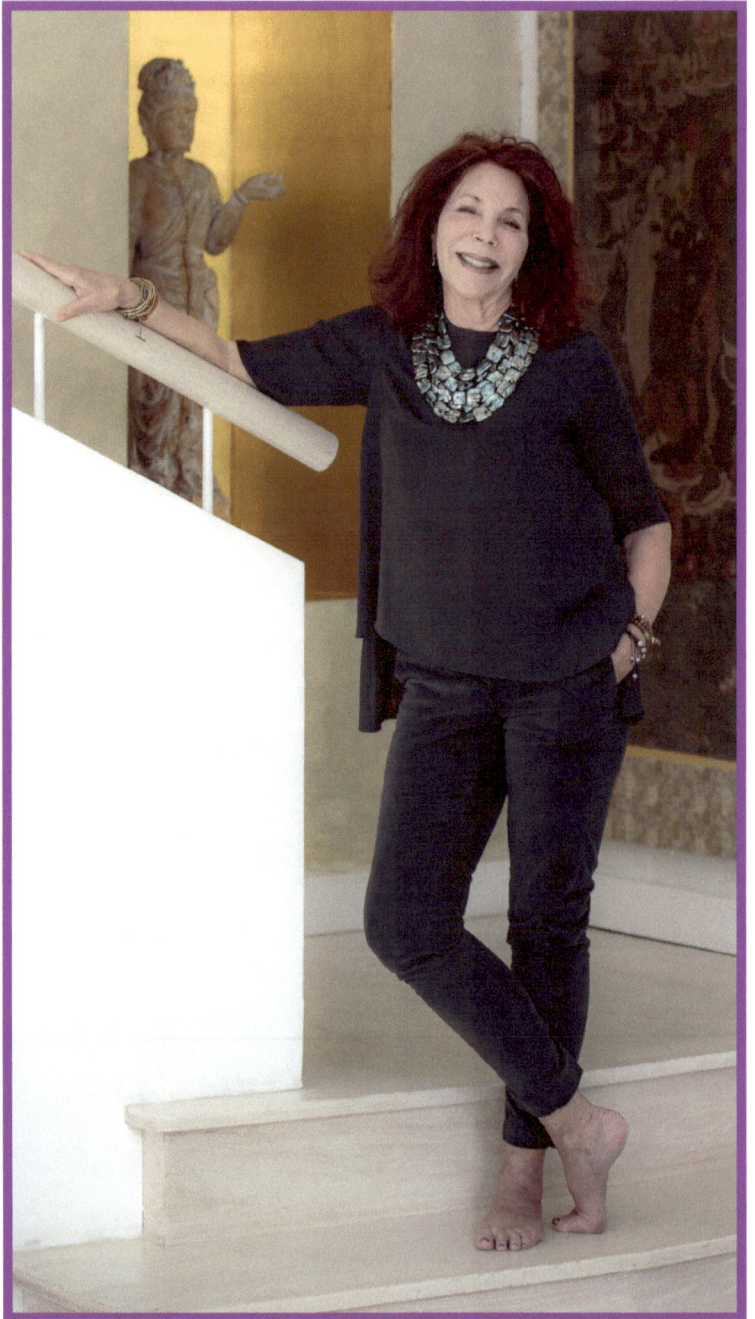

# Name: Marcia Wilson
## Age: 76

Started her personal training with me at the age of 48.
We have been together for a total of **28 years.**

For more than 40 years, Marcia Wilson helped build the brand that was Daffy's, the iconic off-price retailer of clothing and home accessories. Known for its unbeatable bargains, unique merchandise mix and offbeat ads, Daffy's was an innovative pioneer in the retail industry.

In 2013, Marcia founded FORME Enterprises, a creative consulting consortium focused on merchandising and marketing.

*"Exercising these many years
has provided me the sustenance to stay sane
in this insane world
(and fit into my clothes!)"*

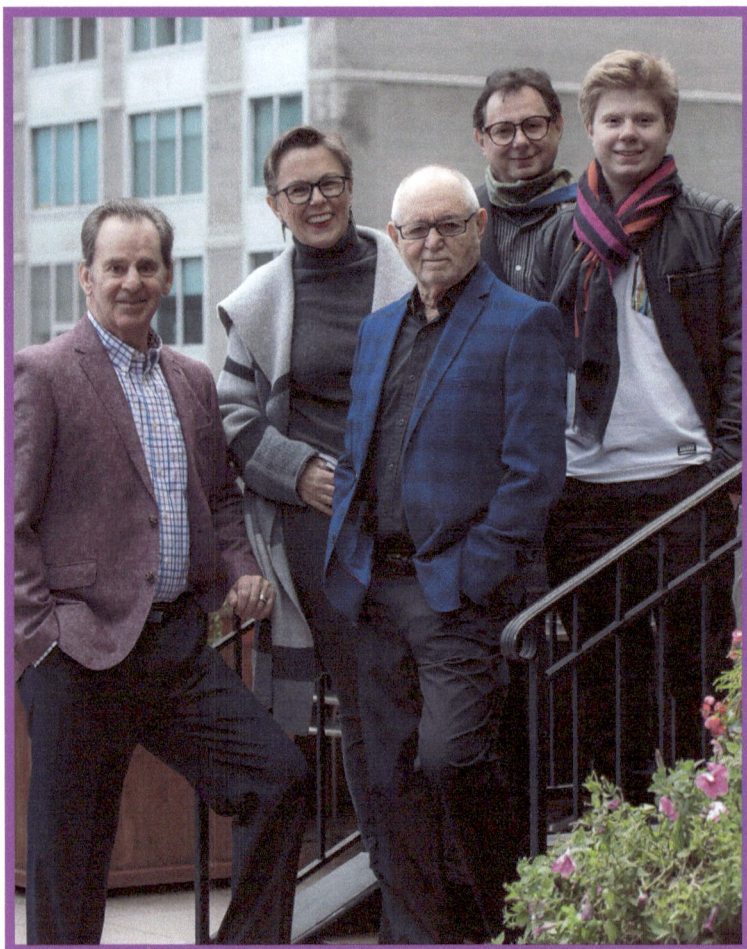

**Left to right:**
Randall Corwin, Susie Lang, Alec Berzack, Gary Berzack,
Maxwell Berzack

# Generations

## Name: Alec Berzack
## Age: 87

### *(Father, Husband, Grandfather)*

Started his personal training with me at the age of 66.
We have been together for a total of **21 years
and counting...**

Born in 1934 in Johannesburg, South Africa, I have been
fortunate to travel a great deal and to have an amazing life.
I am a father *(pretty good I am told)*, a grandfather *(loved)*,
husband *(twice)*, businessman *(pretty successful)*, aviator
*(no crashes)*, horseman *(quite a few falls)*, author *(fiction)*,
golfer *(lousy)*, made money *(lots)*. I have looked after my
body *(keeping fit)* and eating healthy foods *(mostly)*. I have
absorbed wisdom from many *(older and wiser)*. I am still
willing to learn from others (*even though mostly younger
than I am)*. I do not think the past was better–I think now is
the best time of my life.

> *"When 'old age' arrives
> I want to be fit to greet it!"*

# Name: Susie Lang
# Age: 64

## *(Wife, Mother, Grandmother)*

Started her personal training with me at the age of 48.
We have been together for a total of **16 years
and counting...**

Susie is many things and a lover of life! She's a practicing
psychotherapist, a professional photographer, a humanitarian,
a traveler, a wife, an honorary mother, a step-mother, a
grandmother, a sister, a daughter, a good friend to have,
a golfer, and a former dressage rider.

*"I'm learning to find my way in life.
If I can pay attention to myself through my body,
my heart, my mind, my emotions and
my inner-self, I have a chance of making it
into older age with knowledge, integrity, wisdom,
maturity, experience, freedom and inner peace.
I aim to be physically, mentally, emotionally and
spiritually strong to find my own balance."*

# Name: Gary Berzack
# Age: 58

## *(Son, Father)*

Started his personal training with me at the age of 35.
We have been together for a total of **23 years
and counting...**

Gary is a CTO/COO of eTribeca LLC. Active in WiFi and video
conferencing technologies and their practical applications.

*"Consistent exercise helps me to deal
with the ups and downs of life."*

# Name: Randall D. Corwin
# Age: 70
## *(Son-in-Law)*

Started his personal training with me at the age of 53.
We have been together for a total of **17 years
and counting...**

Randy is a Tax Accountant who received his Masters of Law
degree in taxation from NYU Law School. He held a senior
financial position for many years with a very large private
company.

*"I've lived an active life and wish
to continue living that way."*

**Exercise. Why?**

# Name: Maxwell Berzack
## Age: 20

*(Son, Grandson)*

Started his personal training with me at the tender age of 8. We have been together for a total of **12 years and counting...**

Max is currently attending college at Temple University in Philadelphia.

*"I work out not only because it keeps me healthy, but it helps me think clearer and express myself in more positive ways."*

# What I am *most* aware of...

is
how much
I don't
know.

To be continued...

# About the Author

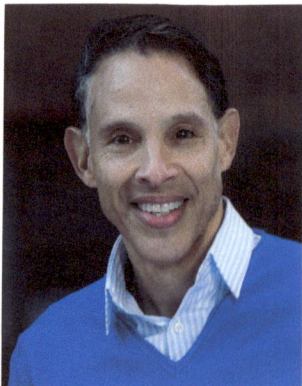

At the age of 14 I began my gymnastics training. Devoting 7 years–four years under Renville Duncan-gymnast, dancer, actor who received the Professor de Gymnastique in Romania, and three years under Abraham Grossfeld, two time Olympian and Head Coach of the 1984 Olympic Games Mens Gold Medal Winning Gymnastics team. I received my B.S. in Physical Education in 1986 from Southern Connecticut State University in New Haven.

I have worked as a personal trainer for the YWCA, Jack Lalanne Health Clubs, the New York Health and Racquet Club, Printing House, and Sports Training Institute. I have also trained privately in the Hamptons. I was a student of the Chinese Kung-Fu Wu-Su Association and a student of Grandmaster Alan Lee for a total of 28 years.

At the age of 24 I started my first private personal training business in a studio apartment. In 1990 at age 25 I opened Fitness Results Inc. at 137 Fifth Avenue in New York City.

With philosophy and medicine on one side and the Warrior and Olympic Games on the other, **Ancient Greece** was my inspiration. This was my role model and where my personal beliefs for a Holistic Health Culture lie, the belief that a human being needs to be touched by all the arts in order to be truly healthy: exercise, nutrition, meditation, music, dance, art work, plants and animals. Fitness Results was not perfect by design, but a laboratory that was based on the following principles:

**Holisticity:** no one piece is greater than the whole; each person is a company unto themselves.

**Integration:** of gender, race, techniques and appearance was encouraged.

**Tolerance:** everyone must respect each others differences and above all the space and others around you.

Instructors at the studio were 100% freelance. There were no memberships and no set work schedules for practitioners, and the cost of the session was determined by the practitioner, not the studio.

I never wanted the studio to be limited by my limitations.

The studio had practitioners proficient in Personal Training, Yoga, Pilates, Gyrotonics, Martial Arts and Dance, Chi-Kung, longevity training, acupuncture, massage therapy, Shiatsu, Reiki, Tibetan and Ayurvedic medicine as well as Quantum Bio Feedback.

Over the studio's 25 years I experienced two recessions, and the loss of four immediate relatives. Difficult lessons learned in overcoming obstacles. At the time I lacked experience in business as well as in life.

I continue to work in NYC as a personal trainer in a one-to-one fashion doing what I love most: **Teaching.** I believe my purpose in this life is to both give and receive through teaching.

# Acknowledgements

To my grandparents, my truest heroes whose unconditional love, guidance and sacrifice, laid the foundation for my happiness, self confidence and personal feeling of security.

To my mother, who gave me life. Your quiet grace, steady love, strength and perseverance, provided me with a blueprint on how to navigate through life's many obstacles.

Dad, the day you took me as your son and gave me your last name, I became not a bastard son, but the luckiest son on earth.

To my sisters, brothers, aunts, uncles, nieces, nephews and cousins I hit the jackpot in life's lottery when I was given you for my family.

Dearest clientele, you have provided me with a broad canvas to express my ideas and fulfill my dreams as a teacher, and I am forever grateful.

Friends and teachers who I have encountered along the way, thank you for imparting your wisdom, kindness and generosity and allowing me to share in your life.

# Credits

## Photography

Susie Lang

## Design

Jeffrey Shammah with Gloria Gregurovich